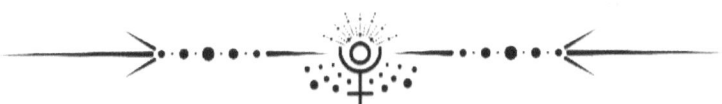

Pluto in Aquarius

Revolutionary Pathways to Health, Healing, and Human Evolution

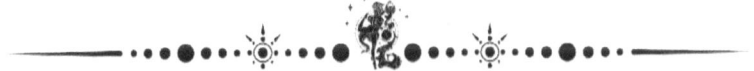

Cynthia Reneé Sumpter

Table of Contents

The Ethical Evolution: Redefining Wellness in the Age of Pluto and Aquarius Exploring the moral and philosophical dimensions of rapid medical and technological advancements.

Collective Healing: Aquarius' Vision of Unity Emphasizing the role of community and shared responsibility in achieving holistic health.

Pluto in Aquarius in the First House: Personal Transformation and Vitality Redefined Exploring the impact of Pluto in Aquarius on self-image, physical health, and individuality.

Pluto in Aquarius in the Second House: Financial Wellness and Nutritional Balance Addressing the connection between resources, values, and maintaining physical and mental health.

Pluto in Aquarius in the Third House: Nervous System and Cognitive Evolution The role of Pluto in Aquarius in enhancing communication, mental agility, and managing stress.

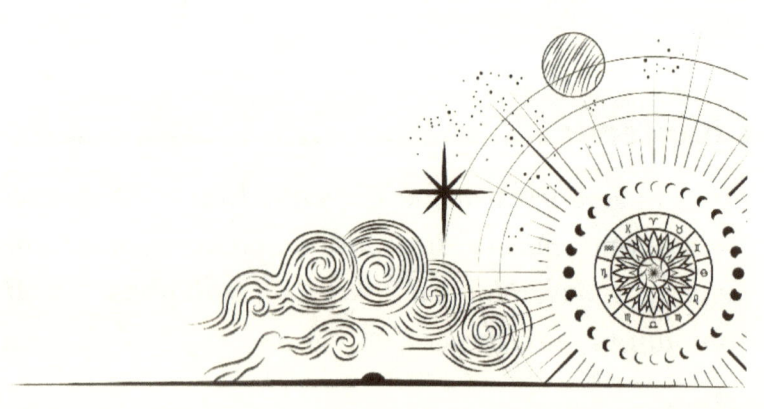

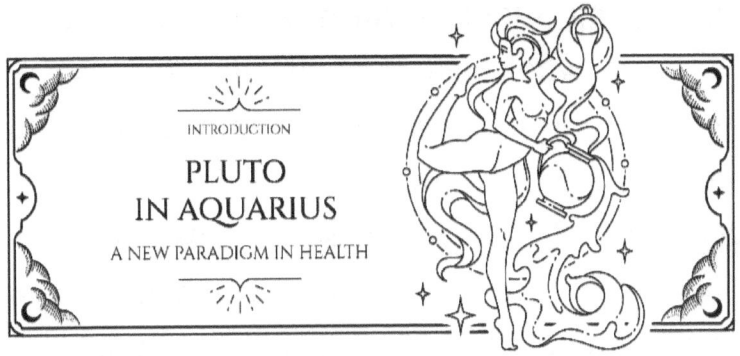

INTRODUCTION

The celestial shift of Pluto into Aquarius marks the dawn of a new era. One where the transformative power of this distant yet potent planet fuses with the forward-thinking energy of the Water Bearer. As humanity steps into this revolutionary age, we are presented with both profound challenges and extraordinary opportunities for growth, particularly in the realm of health and well-being.

Pluto, the harbinger of deep transformation, rules the processes of death, rebirth, and renewal. It is the planet of profound change, unearthing hidden truths and urging us to confront what lies beneath the surface. In Aquarius, a sign associated with innovation, technology, community, and the collective good, Pluto's energy takes on a futuristic lens. Together, they signify a period of groundbreaking medical advancements, shifts in societal health paradigms, and an increased focus on holistic approaches to healing.

This book explores the implications of Pluto's transit through Aquarius on physical, mental, and emotional health. It delves into the potential health challenges that may arise during this transformative period, such as those linked to the nervous system, circulatory issues, and stress induced by rapid societal changes. But more importantly, it highlights the remedies, both ancient and cutting-edge, that align with this cosmic energy— empowering individuals to navigate this epoch with resilience and grace.

From the rise of integrative medicine to the resurgence of communal healing practices, Pluto in Aquarius invites us to redefine health not just as the absence of illness, but as a harmonious balance of body, mind, and spirit within the context of an interconnected world. This book provides insights into how this planetary transit can catalyze personal and collective healing by embracing innovation while staying rooted in timeless wisdom.

Whether you are an astrologer, a holistic health practitioner, or simply someone seeking to understand the cosmic forces shaping our future, this guide offers a comprehensive exploration of Pluto's transformative journey through Aquarius. It is both a map and a compass, designed to help you unlock the healing potential of this profound astrological alignment and harness its energy for your well-being and evolution.

Welcome to a journey of discovery, empowerment, and transformation. Welcome to the era of Pluto in Aquarius.

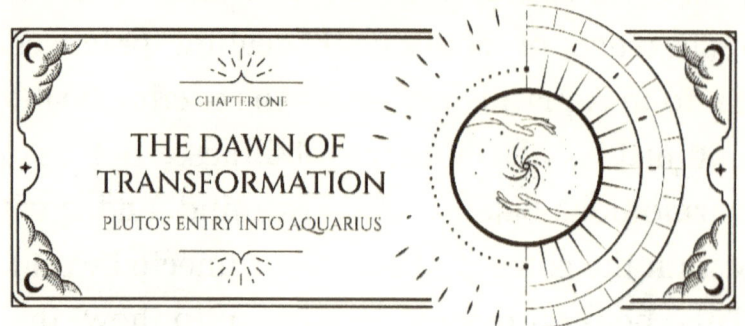

CHAPTER ONE

THE DAWN OF
TRANSFORMATION

PLUTO'S ENTRY INTO AQUARIUS

Chapter 1

The Dawn of Transformation: Pluto's Entry into Aquarius

Pluto's transition into Aquarius heralds a period of profound transformation—both on a personal and collective level. As the planet of regeneration, Pluto pushes humanity to confront the hidden depths of our existence, bringing to light the truths that have long been suppressed. In Aquarius, the sign of innovation, technology, and community, these revelations take on a futuristic and egalitarian focus.

This chapter explores the astrological symbolism of Pluto and Aquarius, delving into how their interplay will reshape our world. Pluto's presence here signals an era where old systems are dismantled, making way for groundbreaking discoveries and unconventional solutions, particularly in the field of health and wellness. From the adoption of cutting-edge medical technologies to the rise of global cooperation in tackling public health challenges, the potential for revolutionary change is immense.

Aquarius' association with the nervous system and circulatory health highlights specific areas of focus during this transit. As stress levels increase due to rapid societal shifts, it becomes imperative to understand and address the physical and emotional tolls of change. This chapter introduces the themes of holistic health and community-driven healing that will be explored throughout the book, emphasizing the importance of balance and adaptation in navigating Pluto's transformative energy.

Pluto's influence often manifests as a crisis, compelling individuals and societies to evolve. However, within these challenges lies the promise of rebirth. As we step into this new era, humanity is called to embrace innovation while staying grounded in the wisdom of the past. This delicate balance between progress and tradition will define our journey through Pluto's transit in Aquarius, setting the stage for the transformative themes discussed in the chapters ahead.

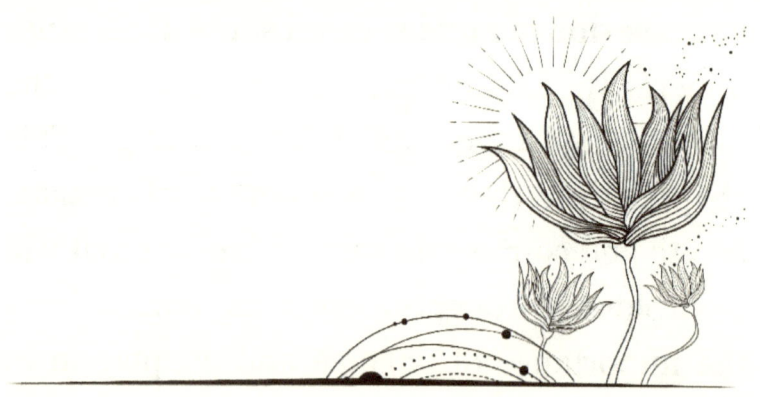

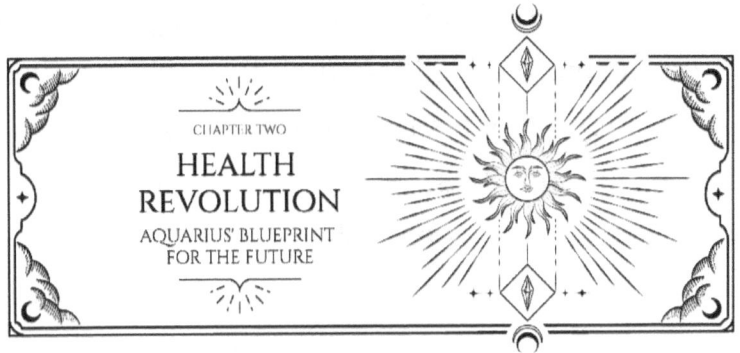

Chapter 2

Health Revolution: Aquarius' Blueprint for the Future

As Pluto's transformative energy aligns with Aquarius' futuristic vision, the way we approach health is set to undergo a profound evolution. This chapter explores the innovative possibilities that emerge when these forces converge, illuminating the ways technology, community, and holistic practices are redefining our understanding of wellness.

Aquarius, ruled by Uranus, thrives on innovation and disruption of the status quo. In the realm of health, this energy brings groundbreaking advancements in medical technology, from precision medicine to AI-driven diagnostics. Personalized healthcare, biohacking, and wearable health devices are just a few examples of how technology will revolutionize the way we monitor, treat, and maintain our physical and mental well-being during Pluto's transit.

Equally significant is Aquarius' focus on the collective and the importance of community-driven health initiatives. The rise of shared health resources, global cooperation in combating diseases, and the adoption of open-access medical research reflect the humanitarian spirit of Aquarius. This period encourages collaboration across borders and disciplines, fostering a united approach to tackling global health challenges.

On a more personal level, the Aquarian emphasis on the nervous system underscores the importance of managing stress, maintaining mental clarity, and enhancing resilience. Techniques such as mindfulness, meditation, and biofeedback, combined with ancient practices like acupuncture and energy healing, will gain renewed importance as people seek balance in an increasingly fast-paced world.

This chapter also delves into the ethical considerations that accompany these advancements. As technology becomes more integrated into healthcare, questions of privacy, access, and equality come to the forefront. Aquarius' egalitarian ethos challenges us to ensure that these innovations benefit all, rather than creating further divides.

Ultimately, Pluto in Aquarius offers an opportunity to redefine health as a harmonious integration of body, mind, and spirit. By embracing both the technological and the timeless, we can create a future where wellness is not merely about curing diseases but fostering a holistic state of balance and vitality for individuals and communities alike. This chapter lays the groundwork for understanding the revolutionary health paradigms that will unfold in the chapters to come.

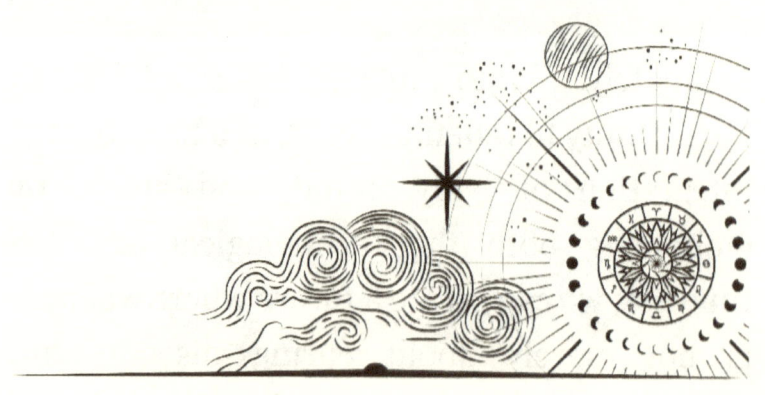

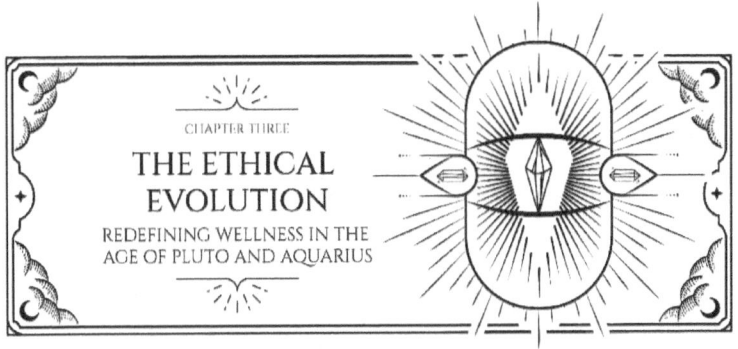

Chapter 3

The Ethical Evolution: Redefining Wellness in the Age of Pluto and Aquarius

As Pluto's transformative journey through Aquarius continues, it ushers in not only technological advancements but also profound ethical questions about the future of health and wellness. This chapter delves into the moral and philosophical dimensions of this transit, examining how society must balance innovation with compassion, equity, and responsibility.

One of the defining features of Aquarius is its commitment to the collective good. This ethos challenges us to ensure that medical breakthroughs, such as gene editing, advanced AI diagnostics, and regenerative therapies, are accessible to all. The risk of creating disparities in healthcare becomes a critical concern as we navigate this period of rapid progress. How can we democratize access to these innovations while avoiding the pitfalls of elitism and exclusion?

Aquarius' focus on technology also raises questions about the limits of human intervention. With advancements like brain-machine interfaces and AI-enhanced treatments, humanity faces a critical juncture: how far should we go in integrating technology into the human body and mind? This chapter explores the philosophical implications of these advancements, including the potential loss of autonomy, the impact on mental health, and the ethical considerations surrounding enhancement versus healing.

At the heart of this ethical evolution lies the need to redefine wellness. Pluto in Aquarius encourages us to move beyond traditional definitions of health and disease, urging us to consider well-being as a dynamic interplay between the individual, community, and environment. This chapter introduces the concept of "planetary health," emphasizing the interconnectedness of human health with ecological sustainability. It explores how environmental degradation, climate change, and resource scarcity will shape global health outcomes during this era.

Ultimately, this chapter calls for a values-driven approach to innovation—one that prioritizes humanity and compassion over profit and power. It underscores the importance of fostering dialogue between scientists, healthcare professionals, ethicists, and communities to create a future where advancements in health and wellness align with the greater good. By integrating ethical considerations into the framework of progress, Pluto in Aquarius can guide humanity toward a more just, equitable, and harmonious future.

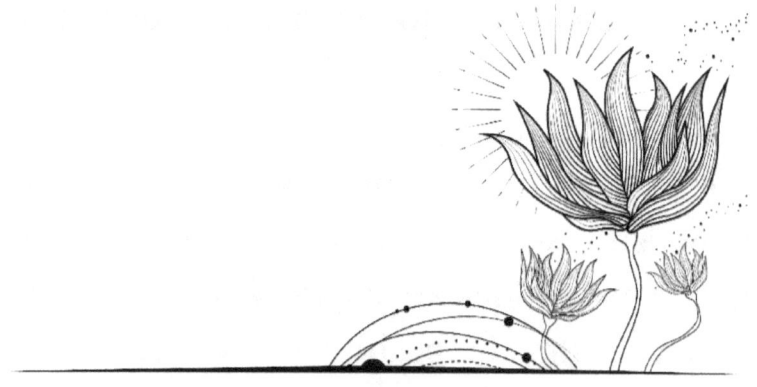

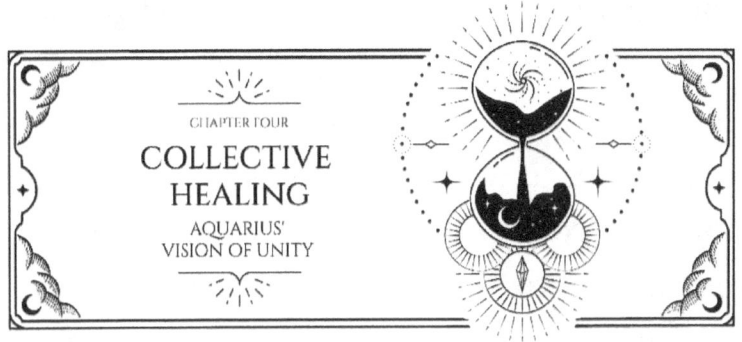

CHAPTER FOUR

COLLECTIVE
HEALING

AQUARIUS'
VISION OF UNITY

Chapter 4

Collective Healing: Aquarius' Vision of Unity

As Pluto's transformative energy continues to reshape societal structures, Aquarius' influence underscores the importance of unity and collective action in achieving holistic health. This chapter focuses on the ways in which collaboration and community-driven initiatives can redefine health and well-being, fostering an interconnected approach to healing.

Aquarius thrives in spaces of shared purpose and collective progress. This ethos invites us to move away from isolated, individualistic approaches to wellness, embracing instead the power of community. From grassroots health movements to global collaborations in disease prevention, the spirit of Aquarius urges humanity to act as one, recognizing that the health of one impacts the health of all.

Key to this collective healing is the resurgence of traditional practices that emphasize communal care. Indigenous healing rituals, group therapies, and cooperative health models are making a return as people seek meaningful connections in their pursuit of well-being. This chapter explores how these practices are being integrated with modern advancements, creating a bridge between ancient wisdom and contemporary science.

Additionally, this chapter delves into the potential of technology to facilitate collective healing. Telemedicine, online support groups, and global health databases are transforming the way people connect and collaborate on health issues. The democratization of health information and resources is breaking down barriers, enabling individuals across the globe to access care and support.

However, this vision of unity is not without challenges. Societal divides, inequities in resource distribution, and cultural differences can hinder progress. Aquarius' energy calls for compassion and understanding, encouraging humanity to embrace diversity while working toward shared goals. By fostering inclusivity and breaking down systemic barriers, collective healing becomes not just a possibility but a reality.

As this chapter concludes, it emphasizes that the path to collective healing is one of shared responsibility. The interconnectedness of human health, social structures, and the environment requires a holistic approach that prioritizes the well-being of all. By aligning with Aquarius' vision of unity, we can harness Pluto's transformative power to create a healthier, more harmonious world.

Pluto in Aquarius in Each House

Pluto represents transformation, regeneration, and power, often associated with profound and intense energy. It governs cycles of destruction and rebirth, making it a planet of deep change.

Aquarius is an air sign ruled by Uranus (and traditionally Saturn). It governs the circulatory system, lower legs, and ankles, as well as the nervous system. Aquarius energy often connects with innovation, rebellion, and humanitarian ideals.

When Pluto occupies Aquarius, it may indicate a unique and powerful transformation in these areas of health. Individuals with this placement may experience sudden breakthroughs in their health patterns or may be drawn to unconventional healing methods.

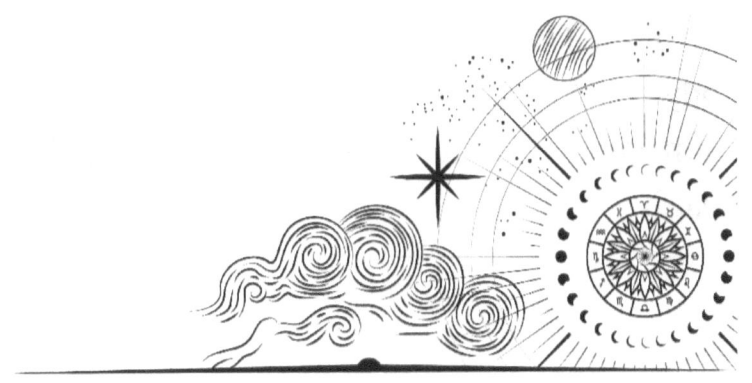

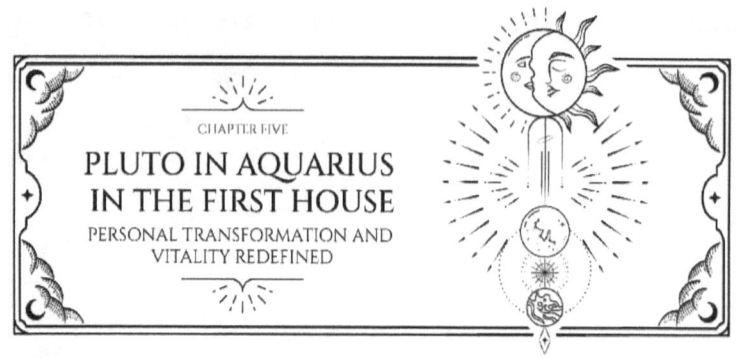

Chapter 5

First House: Personal Transformation and Vitality Redefined

Exploring the impact of Pluto in Aquarius on self-image, physical health, and individuality. The First House represents the self, physical body, and outward appearance. It is deeply connected to vitality and overall physical health.

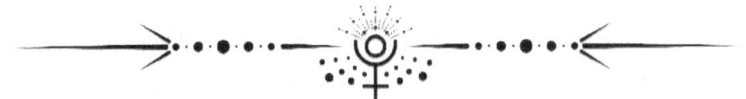

HEALTH IMPLICATIONS

Physical Sensitivity

The circulatory system and nervous system are areas of focus. You might be prone to issues like varicose veins, poor circulation, or nerve-related conditions (e.g., spasms, restless legs, or tingling sensations in the lower limbs).

Pluto's influence suggests that such conditions could arise during intense periods of stress or transformation in life.

Rebirth Through Health

Pluto's transformative energy means that even if health challenges arise, you have an incredible capacity to heal and regenerate. This placement often brings significant life changes through health crises or breakthroughs.

Mental Health and Energy Levels

Pluto in Aquarius suggests a highly active mental state that may lead to burnout or exhaustion if not managed properly. It's important to balance mental overactivity with relaxation techniques.

Unconventional Healing

This placement draws you toward alternative or futuristic methods of health management. Technologies or therapies like biofeedback, energy healing, or advancements in medical science could resonate with you.

Psychosomatic Connections

Pluto's transformative nature often reveals that emotional or psychological shifts manifest in physical health. Awareness and management of stress are crucial.

Potential for Long-Term Vitality

With care, individuals with this placement can experience vitality and strength through periods of personal growth, especially if they embrace Aquarian ideals of progressive, innovative thinking in their approach to health.

SUGGESTIONS FOR WELLNESS

Physical Activities
Engage in regular physical activities that promote circulation, like yoga, swimming, or walking.

Stress Management
Explore stress management techniques such as meditation or breathwork to support the nervous system.

Unique Practices
Consider integrating unconventional health practices aligned with Aquarian principles, like acupuncture or futuristic medical technologies.

Grounding Practice

Stay grounded with routine and self-care to counteract potential emotional intensity brought by Pluto.

Herbs

Ginseng for vitality, chamomile for calming the nervous system, and nettle for supporting circulation.

Gemstones

Carnelian for energy and vitality, hematite for grounding, and clear quartz for overall balance.

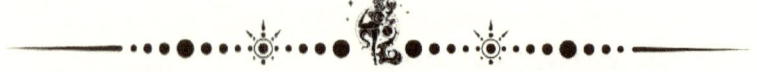

This placement speaks to the profound power of personal transformation through physical and mental health journeys.

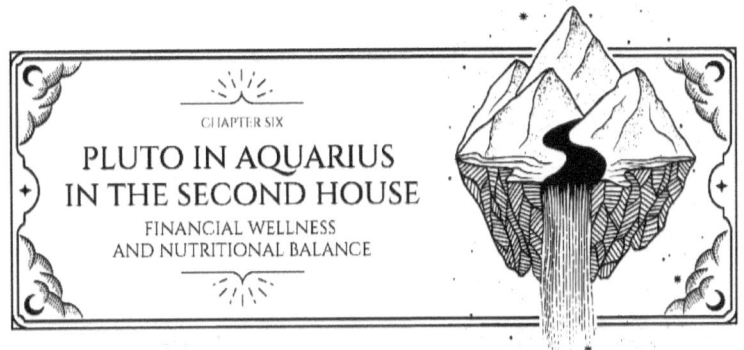

Chapter 6

Pluto in Aquarius in the Second House: Financial Wellness and Nutritional Balance

Addressing the connection between resources, values, and maintaining physical and mental health. Pluto in Aquarius in the Second House carries specific health implications due to the connection between Pluto, Aquarius, and the Second House. Here's a detailed breakdown:

Pluto governs transformation, intensity, and regeneration, bringing deep shifts in the areas it touches.

Aquarius, an air sign, rules the circulatory system, lower legs, ankles, and the nervous system. It also symbolizes progressive, innovative energy.

Second House (Resources and Values)

The Second House is traditionally associated with values, resources, self-worth, and material possessions. When related to health, it emphasizes nutrition, physical resources (the body as a resource), and how we sustain and nurture ourselves.

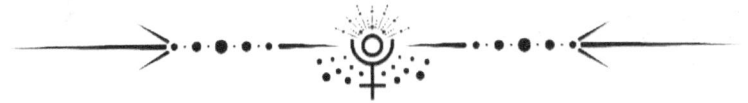

HEALTH IMPLICATIONS

Metabolic Sensitivity

The Second House relates to sustenance, so Pluto here often indicates an intense relationship with food and nutrition.

You may have periods of extremes: either an obsessive focus on diet and health or neglect of it. Nutritional deficiencies or sensitivities could arise if balance isn't maintained.

Weight and Energy Regulation

Pluto's influence can bring fluctuations in weight or energy levels. Aquarius adds an erratic element, so you might experience times of high energy alternating with periods of fatigue.

Impact of Emotional States on Health

The Second House connects to self-worth. Emotional challenges, particularly related to how you value yourself, might manifest in health concerns like eating disorders, stress-related digestion issues, or even hormonal imbalances.

Circulation and Nervous System

Pluto in Aquarius emphasizes the circulatory system and nervous system. Issues such as poor circulation, varicose veins, or restless legs may stem from unresolved emotional stress or lifestyle imbalances.

Regenerative Healing Potential

Pluto grants a remarkable capacity for regeneration. If health challenges arise, you have the ability to transform and rebuild through focused effort, especially by embracing unconventional or innovative health practices.

Psychological Attachment to Material Resources

Your health might be influenced by your emotional relationship with security and possessions. Anxiety about financial stability or self-worth could manifest physically, affecting your digestion, metabolism, or overall vitality.

SUGGESTIONS FOR WELLNESS

Focus on Balanced Nutrition

Ensure a well-rounded diet rich in nutrients to support metabolism and circulation. Avoid extreme diets or habits.

Stress Management

Since emotional states can influence your health, practices like journaling, therapy, or meditation can help maintain inner balance.

Innovative Health Practices

Explore modern or unconventional health solutions. Technologies or therapies that align with Aquarian energy, such as biofeedback, intermittent fasting, or energy medicine, might resonate with you.

Physical Activity for Circulation

Activities that promote circulation, like walking, yoga, or swimming, can mitigate Aquarius-related challenges with the legs and ankles.

Build Self-Worth Through Inner Work

Address any issues related to self-esteem or financial stress. Developing a strong sense of self-worth can improve both mental and physical well-being.

Watch for Signs of Stress-Related Disorders

Pay attention to symptoms like digestive issues, fatigue, or circulatory concerns and address them promptly with a combination of traditional and alternative methods.

Herbs
Dandelion root for detoxification, cinnamon for metabolic balance, and ginger for digestive health.

Gemstones
Jade for prosperity and well-being, tiger's eye for self-worth, and citrine for motivation.

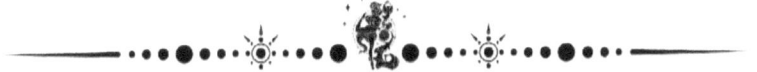

This placement invites you to cultivate a healthy relationship with your physical resources (your body), emotional security, and material possessions. Pluto's transformative power can help you grow stronger through health challenges, ultimately leading to a more balanced and fulfilling life.

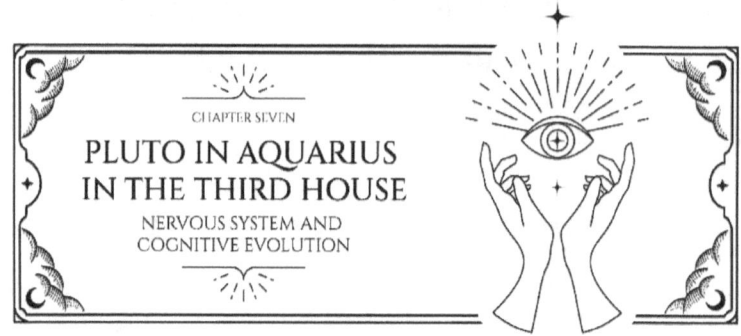

CHAPTER SEVEN

PLUTO IN AQUARIUS
IN THE THIRD HOUSE

NERVOUS SYSTEM AND
COGNITIVE EVOLUTION

Chapter 7

Pluto in Aquarius in the Third House: Nervous System and Cognitive Evolution

The role of Pluto in Aquarius in enhancing communication, mental agility, and managing stress. Pluto in Aquarius in the Third House brings unique health implications influenced by the themes of Pluto, Aquarius, and the Third House. Here's an in-depth exploration:

Pluto signifies transformation, intensity, and deep regeneration, impacting the areas it governs with profound energy.

Aquarius governs the circulatory system, lower legs, ankles, and the nervous system. Its air element also links it to mental and intellectual processes.

Third House (Communication and Mind)

The Third House rules communication, the mind, learning, short-distance travel, and close relatives (like siblings). When connected to health, it highlights mental health, respiratory health, and the nervous system.

Health Implications

Mental Overactivity

The Third House, combined with Pluto's intensity and Aquarius's mental agility, can result in overthinking, mental exhaustion, or nervous tension. This could lead to issues like headaches, anxiety, or insomnia.

Respiratory and Throat Concerns

The Third House governs the lungs and respiratory system, so there could be a tendency toward asthma, bronchitis, or other conditions linked to breathing. Aquarius may amplify this with stress-induced symptoms.

Stress and Nervous System Sensitivity

Pluto in Aquarius in this house suggests heightened sensitivity in the nervous system. Symptoms like nervous tics, restlessness, or stress-related disorders may arise during emotionally charged times.

Impact of Communication on Health

Emotional suppression or difficulty expressing yourself might manifest as physical symptoms. For example, unresolved tensions with siblings or close relatives could contribute to mental stress or psychosomatic illnesses.

Sudden Health Episodes

With Aquarius, health concerns may arise suddenly and unpredictably but often respond well to innovative or unconventional treatment methods.

Potential for Mental Regeneration

Pluto offers incredible regenerative power. If mental or physical health challenges occur, you possess the capacity to transform your habits and mindset, emerging stronger and more resilient.

Suggestions for Wellness

Stress Management Techniques
Prioritize practices that calm the mind and nervous system, such as mindfulness meditation, yoga, or journaling.

Breathing Exercises
Incorporate breathwork or pranayama to support respiratory health and mental clarity.

Healthy Communication
Address any lingering conflicts with siblings or close relatives through open and honest dialogue. Consider therapy if communication patterns feel blocked.

Physical Movement for Circulation
Regular physical activity, like walking, swimming, or even dance, can help alleviate

tension and promote circulation, especially in the lower body (Aquarius influence).

Unconventional Healing
Explore alternative health modalities such as acupuncture, sound therapy, or biofeedback to address nervous system imbalances.

Limit Overstimulation
Reduce exposure to excessive mental stimulation (e.g., screen time, social media) to prevent burnout and maintain focus.

Herbs
Peppermint for clarity, lemon balm for calming mental overactivity, and rosemary for memory support.

Gemstones
Blue lace agate for communication, fluorite for mental clarity, and amethyst for intuition.

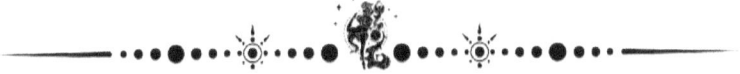

With Pluto in Aquarius in the Third House, your mental and emotional health are closely tied to your physical well-being. Overthinking, unresolved emotional tension, or poor communication habits may manifest as physical symptoms, particularly in the respiratory and nervous systems. However, Pluto's transformative power allows you to regenerate and heal profoundly by embracing balance and innovation in your approach to health and communication.

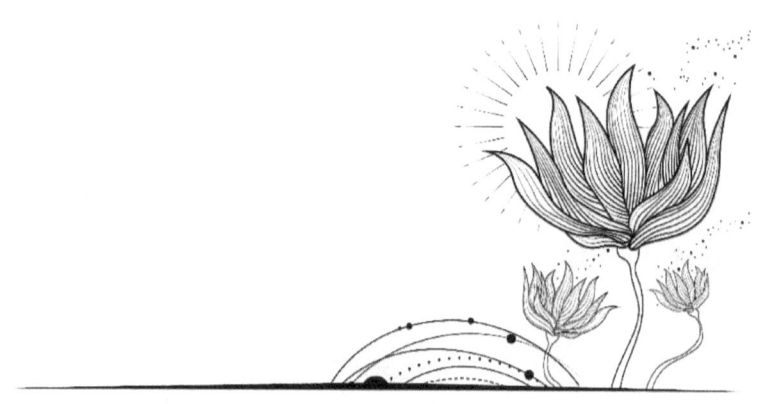

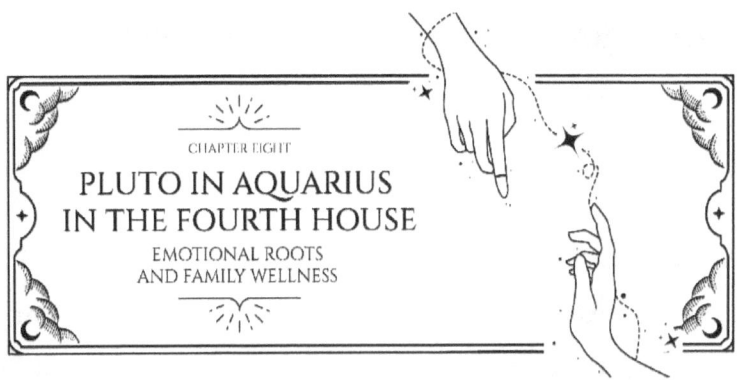

Chapter 8

Pluto in Aquarius in the Fourth House: Emotional Roots and Family Wellness

Focusing on the influence of home, ancestry, and emotional stability on health. Pluto in Aquarius in the Fourth House brings a unique blend of transformative energy to areas connected to home, family, and emotional foundations. This placement has notable health implications tied to emotional well-being and how you connect with your roots.

Pluto governs transformation, power, and regeneration, influencing deep, often hidden processes of growth.

Aquarius, as an air sign, rules the circulatory system, lower legs, ankles, and the nervous system. It also represents innovative, future-focused, and sometimes detached energy.

Fourth House (Home and Emotional Foundation)

The Fourth House relates to home, family, emotional security, and the subconscious. It governs your foundational well-being, including the effects of childhood and family dynamics on health.

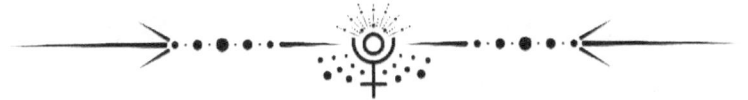

Health Implications

Psychosomatic Health

Emotional challenges stemming from family dynamics or unresolved childhood issues may manifest as physical symptoms. For example, suppressed emotions could contribute to digestive issues or nervous tension.

Circulatory and Nervous System Sensitivity

Aquarius emphasizes the nervous system and circulation. Stress from family or home-related matters might result in poor circulation, tension in the legs and ankles, or nervous disorders.

Emotional Stress and Its Effects

Pluto in the Fourth House suggests that emotional intensity or upheaval in your private life can directly impact your health. You might experience sleep disturbances, anxiety, or chronic fatigue tied to unresolved emotional concerns.

Transformative Healing Through Home and Family

While challenges in your familial relationships may arise, Pluto's influence provides the power for deep emotional healing and renewal. This, in turn, can lead to profound improvements in health.

Tendencies Toward Isolation

Pluto's placement may encourage periods of retreat or isolation, especially during times of stress. While this can be regenerative, prolonged isolation may lead to feelings of detachment or depression, impacting mental and physical health.

Inherited Health Patterns

The Fourth House can indicate inherited traits, including health vulnerabilities. There might be a family history of circulatory or nervous system issues, which you'll need to address proactively.

Suggestions for Wellness

Address Emotional Foundations
Engage in therapy or counseling to explore family dynamics and childhood experiences that may be affecting your emotional and physical well-being.

Create a Healing Environment at Home
Make your home a sanctuary. Introduce calming elements like plants, soft lighting, or healing music to reduce stress.

Breathwork and Grounding Practices
To counteract Aquarius's nervous energy, practice grounding techniques like meditation, breathwork, or yoga.

Nutrition for Emotional Stability
A balanced diet rich in magnesium and omega-3s can support your nervous system and overall mental health

Strengthen Circulation
Engage in activities like walking, cycling, or swimming to enhance blood flow, particularly to the lower body.

Explore Family Healing
Work on improving communication and understanding within your family. Releasing old resentments or patterns can lead to emotional and physical relief.

Herbs
Lavender for relaxation, valerian for emotional stress, and oats for soothing anxiety.

Gemstones
Moonstone for emotional balance, smoky quartz for grounding, and rose quartz for familial harmony.

Pluto in Aquarius in the Fourth House ties your health closely to your emotional and familial well-being. Challenges may arise through stress related to family, home, or childhood memories, often manifesting in the nervous system or circulatory issues. However, Pluto offers profound transformative power, enabling you to heal deeply and create a healthier relationship with your roots, leading to overall wellness and regeneration.

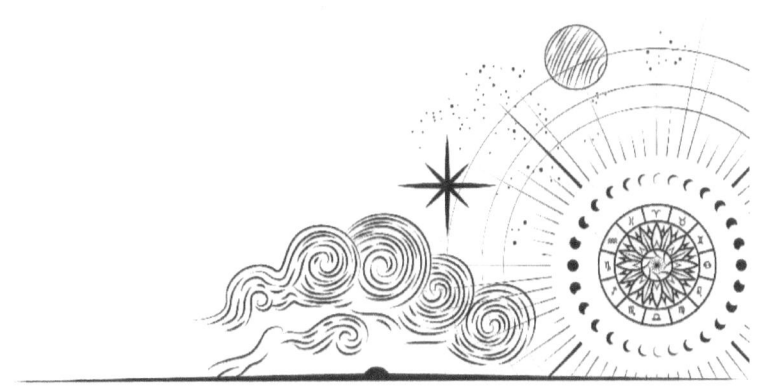

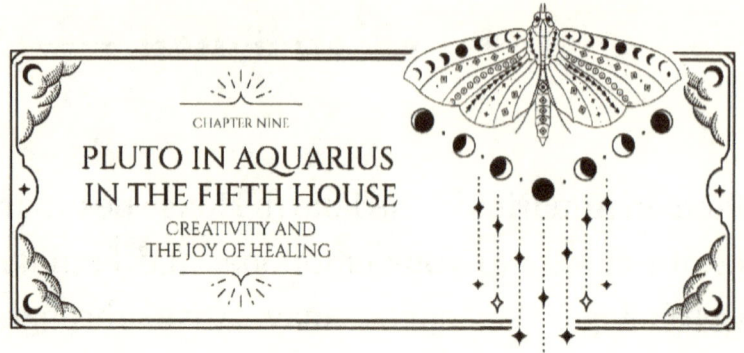

Chapter 9

Pluto in Aquarius in the Fifth House: Creativity and the Joy of Healing

Examining how hobbies, children, and pleasure contribute to holistic well-being. Pluto in Aquarius in the Fifth House combines the transformative energy of Pluto, the innovative spirit of Aquarius, and the creativity and self-expression of the Fifth House. This placement brings notable health implications tied to self-expression, creativity, and the heart.

Pluto symbolizes transformation, power, and regeneration, often working through deep and intense processes of change.

Aquarius, as an air sign, rules the circulatory system, nervous system, lower legs, and ankles. It is futuristic, intellectual, and sometimes detached in its approach.

Fifth House (Creativity and Joy)

The Fifth House governs creativity, self-expression, romance, children, joy, and recreation. It also has ties to the physical heart, spine, and vitality, reflecting how passion and joy influence your health.

HEALTH IMPLICATIONS

Heart Health and Emotional Expression
The Fifth House is associated with the heart, both physically and metaphorically. Pluto's intense energy in this house suggests that suppressed emotions or an inability to express yourself creatively could contribute to heart-related issues or tension in the chest area.

Stress from Overcommitment or Perfectionism
Pluto can intensify your drive for creative or romantic fulfillment. This drive may lead to burnout or stress, especially if you overextend yourself in pursuit of perfection or recognition.

Impact of Joy and Passion on Health
Your overall health may be deeply connected to your ability to experience joy and engage in creative or playful activities. A lack of these can

result in low vitality, fatigue, or even depression.

Sudden Health Challenges

With Aquarius's influence, health challenges may arise suddenly and unpredictably, particularly during emotionally charged periods or moments of creative blockages.

Psychological Ties to Physical Symptoms

Pluto's placement suggests that psychological or emotional struggles related to self-expression, romantic relationships, or children could manifest as physical ailments, particularly affecting the circulatory system or nervous system.

Healing Through Creativity

Pluto's regenerative energy can be channeled through creative outlets, helping to release pent-up emotions and fostering physical and emotional healing.

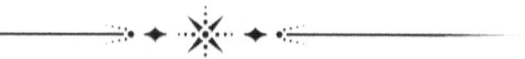

SUGGESTIONS FOR WELLNESS

Heart-Healthy Practices
Prioritize cardiovascular health through regular exercise (like walking, swimming, or dancing) and a heart-healthy diet rich in fruits, vegetables, and omega-3s.

Engage in Creative Expression
Channel Pluto's transformative energy into creative pursuits like art, writing, music, or other hobbies that bring you joy. This can be incredibly therapeutic.

Balance Work and Play
Avoid overcommitting to projects or relationships. Allow yourself time for recreation and relaxation to prevent burnout.

Emotional Release

Practice techniques like journaling, therapy, or breathwork to release suppressed emotions that could be affecting your physical health.

Strengthen the Nervous System

Incorporate practices like meditation, yoga, or tai chi to calm the nervous system and enhance mental clarity.

Mind Romantic and Parental Relationships

Address any tensions in your romantic life or with your children (if applicable). These relationships may have a profound impact on your emotional and physical health.

Herbs

Passionflower for emotional expression, hibiscus for heart health, and holy basil for reducing stress.

Gemstones

Sunstone for joy and creativity, garnet for passion, and ruby for vitality.

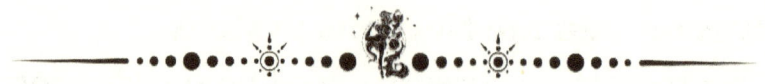

Pluto in Aquarius in the Fifth House highlights the profound connection between health and self-expression. Your vitality thrives when you embrace creativity, joy, and passion. Challenges may arise if emotional or creative outlets are blocked, potentially manifesting in heart-related or nervous system issues. However, Pluto's transformative power empowers you to heal deeply through creative expression and emotional release, leading to greater vitality and well-being.

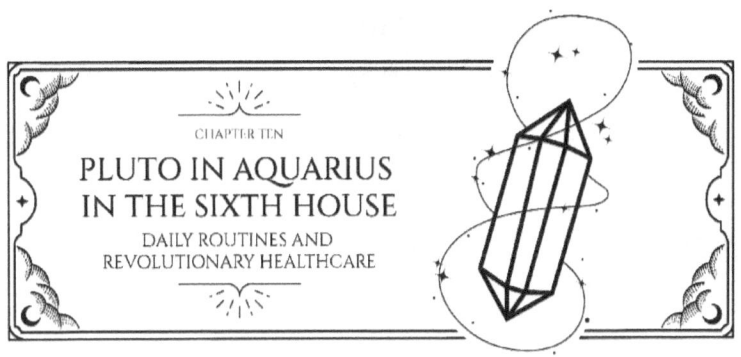

Chapter 10

Pluto in Aquarius in the Sixth House: Daily Routines and Revolutionary Healthcare

Redefining work-life balance, nutrition, and approaches to chronic health conditions. Pluto in Aquarius in the Sixth House strongly influences your health, daily routines, and approach to work and service. This placement highlights transformative potential in health, particularly related to innovation, emotional resilience, and habits.

Pluto represents transformation, intensity, and regeneration, often signaling profound changes and challenges that lead to growth.

Aquarius, an air sign, rules the circulatory system, lower legs, ankles, and the nervous system. It is also associated with progressive, unconventional thinking and innovation.

Sixth House (Health and Routines)

The Sixth House governs health, wellness, daily routines, work, and service. It represents the body as it interacts with lifestyle habits and stress.

This house is directly connected to how you manage your physical health, diet, work environment, and overall well-being.

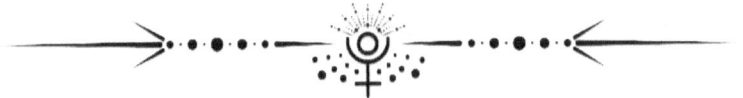

Health Implications

Nervous System Sensitivity

The combination of Pluto's intensity and Aquarius's connection to the nervous system can lead to stress-related disorders, anxiety, or burnout if routines are not balanced. Nervous energy or overwork can amplify these issues.

Circulatory System

Potential issues with circulation, particularly in the lower legs and ankles, might arise. Activities promoting blood flow and movement are essential to maintaining health.

Stress-Driven Health Concerns

Pluto in the Sixth House can bring hidden or long-term health challenges, often tied to stress or unresolved emotional issues. Chronic fatigue, autoimmune disorders, or other conditions may surface during high-pressure periods.

Transformative Healing Potential

This placement gives you the ability to completely regenerate your health and lifestyle after a crisis or health challenge. Embracing innovative or unconventional approaches to wellness can be a turning point.

Obsessive Focus on Health or Routines

Pluto may drive an intense focus on health, fitness, or daily habits, sometimes leading to extremes. While this focus can bring significant improvements, it's crucial to avoid obsessive or rigid behaviors.

Work-Related Health Issues

Stress or dissatisfaction in the workplace can directly impact your physical and mental health. Toxic work environments or overwork may trigger health concerns, particularly related to anxiety or physical exhaustion.

Suggestions for Wellness

Stress Management
Incorporate relaxation techniques like mindfulness, meditation, or yoga to calm the nervous system.

Innovative Health Practices
Consider exploring alternative therapies, such as acupuncture, biofeedback, or advanced medical technology, to address health concerns.

Physical Movement
Regular exercise, particularly activities that stimulate circulation (e.g., walking, swimming, cycling), can help maintain your health and ease tension in the lower body.

Healthy Work-Life Balance

Set boundaries in your work environment to avoid burnout. Ensure your daily routine includes time for rest and self-care.

Nutritional Support

Focus on a nutrient-dense diet to support the nervous system and overall vitality. Include foods rich in magnesium, omega-3s, and antioxidants.

Routine Check-Ups

Since Pluto in the Sixth House can bring hidden health challenges, regular medical check-ups and preventative care are essential.

Herbs

Ashwagandha for adrenal support, lemon balm for calming routines, and turmeric for inflammation.

Gemstones

Green aventurine for healing, jasper for balance, and bloodstone for vitality.

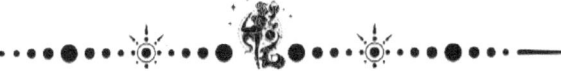

Pluto in Aquarius in the Sixth House connects health and daily routines with transformation and innovation. Challenges may arise through stress, work-life imbalance, or emotional tension, but this placement offers profound regenerative power. By embracing balanced habits and exploring unconventional health solutions, you can achieve lasting wellness and thrive in both your work and personal life.

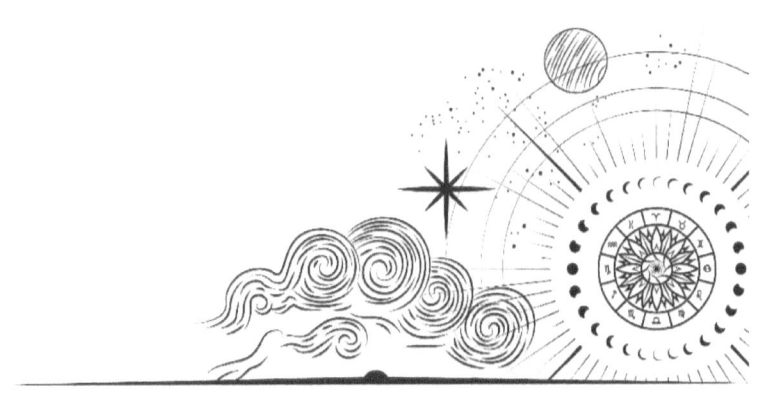

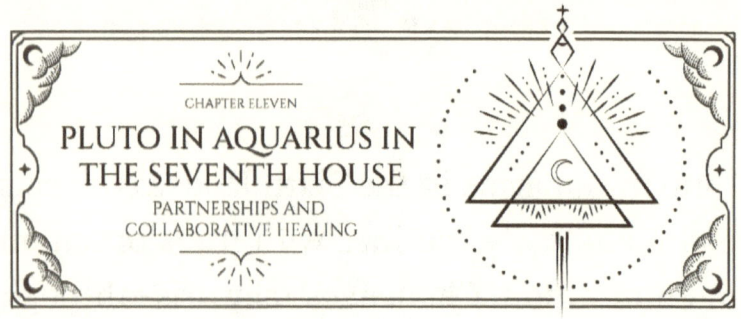

Chapter 11

Pluto in Aquarius in the Seventh House: Partnerships and Collaborative Healing

The impact of relationships and partnerships on mental and emotional wellness. Pluto in Aquarius in the Seventh House places a strong focus on transformation in relationships, partnerships, and how you connect with others. This placement can also reflect health implications tied to emotional dynamics and partnerships.

Pluto represents deep transformation, intensity, and regeneration, often uncovering hidden truths or challenges for growth.

Aquarius, as an air sign, governs the circulatory system, lower legs, ankles, and nervous system. It brings innovation, detachment, and a forward-thinking approach to relationships and health.

Seventh House (Partnerships and Relationships)

The Seventh House rules partnerships, marriage, significant one-on-one relationships, and how you relate to others. It also reflects the balance (or imbalance) you experience in partnerships and how they affect your well-being.

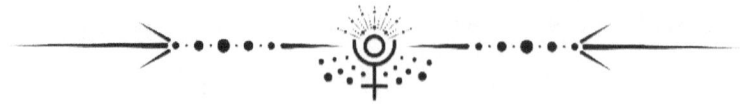

Health Implications

Stress from Relationships

Intense or tumultuous relationships may manifest as physical or mental health challenges. Emotional stress caused by power struggles, betrayal, or manipulation in partnerships could lead to issues like anxiety, insomnia, or nervous tension.

Nervous System Sensitivity

The Aquarius influence highlights the nervous system. Stressful dynamics in your relationships could exacerbate issues such as chronic fatigue, restlessness, or overthinking.

Circulatory Issues

Pluto's transformative energy may bring circulatory problems, particularly in the lower body (legs and ankles), often as a reflection of emotional tension in partnerships.

Psychosomatic Symptoms
Emotional strain from relationships may trigger physical symptoms, particularly in areas associated with Aquarius (nervous system and circulation).

Transformative Healing Through Relationships
Difficult partnerships may serve as catalysts for personal transformation and growth. Healing old wounds and creating healthy emotional boundaries can significantly improve overall well-being.

Dependency or Power Dynamics
Relationships involving control, dependency, or unresolved trauma can drain energy, leading to health imbalances. Learning to establish boundaries is key.

Suggestions for Wellness

Emotional Boundaries
Develop strong boundaries in relationships to protect your emotional and physical health. Address power imbalances early on to avoid stress buildup.

Stress Management
Engage in relaxation techniques such as meditation, yoga, or tai chi to calm the nervous system and maintain emotional equilibrium.

Physical Movement
Activities that promote circulation (e.g., walking, swimming, or stretching) can help alleviate tension, especially in the lower legs and ankles.

Therapeutic Support

Consider therapy or counseling to work through challenges in partnerships. This can help resolve emotional wounds that may be affecting your health.

Innovative Healing Approaches

Explore unconventional or progressive health methods, such as biofeedback, acupuncture, or energy healing, particularly if stress manifests physically.

Work on Self-Empowerment

Focus on personal growth and self-empowerment. Stronger self-confidence can reduce dependency on others and improve overall health.

Herbs

Rose for emotional harmony, chamomile for relational stress, and hawthorn for heart health.

Gemstones

Rhodonite for relationship healing, kunzite for heart connection, and emerald for partnership.

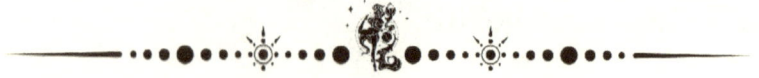

Pluto in Aquarius in the Seventh House, your health is intricately tied to your relationships. Intense or stressful partnerships can impact your emotional and physical well-being, but they also hold the potential for profound transformation and healing. By cultivating healthy boundaries, embracing innovative healing practices, and focusing on emotional resilience, you can create balance in your relationships and achieve overall wellness.

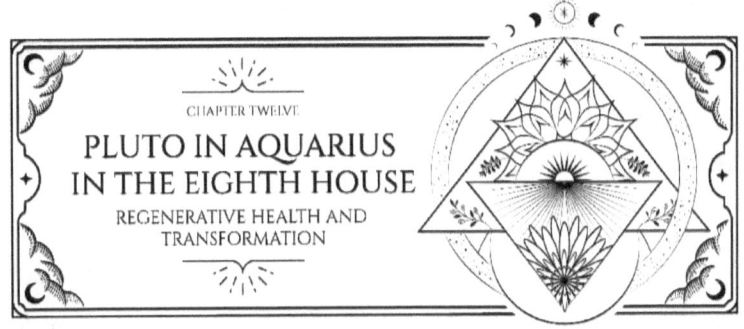

Chapter 12

Pluto in Aquarius in the Eighth House: Regenerative Health and Transformation

Focusing on healing crises, intimacy, and the transformative power of change. Pluto in Aquarius in the Eighth House brings deep, transformative energy to areas related to shared resources, intimacy, power dynamics, and matters of life, death, and rebirth. This placement has profound health implications, often tied to psychological and emotional well-being.

Pluto represents intensity, transformation, and regeneration. Its influence can manifest as deep psychological shifts and a need for renewal.

Aquarius, an air sign, governs the circulatory system, lower legs, ankles, and the nervous system. It is associated with innovation, detachment, and forward-thinking approaches.

Eighth House (Transformation and Shared Resources)

The Eighth House governs themes of transformation, shared resources, intimacy, and hidden aspects of the self. Health concerns in this house are often linked to emotional and psychological undercurrents and may involve crises that lead to profound healing.

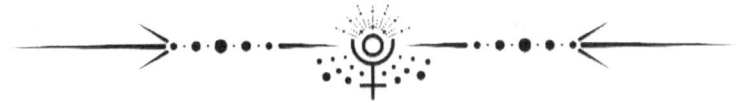

HEALTH IMPLICATIONS

Emotional-Physical Connection
Deep-seated emotions, unresolved traumas, or psychological stress may manifest physically. Symptoms could include nervous system disorders, hormonal imbalances, or issues related to reproductive health.

Regenerative Healing
Pluto's placement in the Eighth House offers remarkable healing potential. You may experience health crises that serve as turning points, leading to profound renewal and transformation.

Circulatory and Nervous System Sensitivity
Aquarius's influence highlights potential vulnerabilities in the circulatory and nervous

systems. Symptoms such as poor circulation, tension in the lower limbs, or stress-related disorders might arise during emotionally intense periods.

Tendency for Extremes
Pluto can bring an all-or-nothing attitude toward health. This may manifest as an intense focus on health practices or neglecting them entirely, depending on emotional states.

Psychosomatic Illnesses
The Eighth House's association with the subconscious means unaddressed emotional wounds or power struggles may lead to psychosomatic conditions.

Innovative Healing Practices
Aquarius's progressive energy suggests you may benefit from alternative or futuristic health modalities, such as energy healing, cutting-edge medical technology, or psychological therapies.

SUGGESTIONS FOR WELLNESS

Address Emotional and Psychological Roots

Explore therapy, counseling, or shadow work to process hidden emotions and traumas. This can prevent emotional stress from manifesting physically.

Innovative Health Approaches

Consider alternative healing modalities, such as acupuncture, biofeedback, or advanced medical treatments that align with Aquarius's futuristic energy.

Support the Nervous System

Engage in practices like yoga, meditation, or breathwork to calm the mind and promote overall well-being.

Hormonal and Reproductive Health

Regular check-ups are essential, particularly for reproductive health or hormonal balance.

Physical Movement for Circulation

Engage in activities that promote blood flow, like walking, swimming, or dance, to support circulation and lower-body health.

Healthy Intimacy

Cultivate trust and emotional depth in intimate relationships. Healthy emotional connections can significantly improve your mental and physical well-being.

Herbs

Skullcap for calming transformations, reishi for regeneration, and yarrow for emotional boundaries.

Gemstones

Obsidian for deep transformation, labradorite for mystical connection, and malachite for healing.

Pluto in Aquarius in the Eighth House emphasizes transformation and healing through emotional, psychological, and physical renewal. Challenges may stem from unresolved traumas or intense emotional dynamics, often manifesting in the circulatory, nervous, or reproductive systems. By embracing innovative health approaches, addressing emotional roots, and fostering deep intimacy, you can harness this placement's transformative potential to achieve profound healing and regeneration.

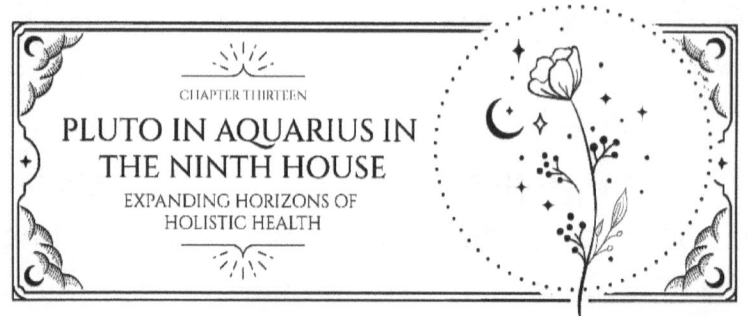

Chapter 13

Pluto in Aquarius in the Ninth House: Expanding Horizons of Holistic Health

Exploring global health practices, spiritual growth, and philosophical shifts in wellness. Pluto in Aquarius in the Ninth House, the themes of transformation, exploration, and intellectual growth significantly influence your health. This placement ties health to belief systems, higher learning, travel, and your connection to broader life philosophies.

Pluto represents transformation, intensity, and the power of renewal, often pushing for deep changes in the areas it touches.

Aquarius, as an air sign, rules the circulatory system, lower legs, ankles, and the nervous system. It also symbolizes forward-thinking, innovation, and detachment.

Ninth House (Beliefs and Expansion)

The Ninth House governs higher education, philosophy, spirituality, long-distance travel, and expanding one's horizons. When connected to health, it often highlights the impact of mindset, spiritual practices, and travel on overall well-being.

HEALTH IMPLICATIONS

Mind-Body Connection
Your beliefs and mindset play a significant role in your health. Negative thought patterns or limiting belief systems may contribute to physical symptoms, particularly in the nervous or circulatory systems.

Stress During Travel
Long-distance travel or disruptions to routine may cause stress, impacting the nervous system or creating tension in the lower body (legs and ankles).

Philosophical Crises and Health
Periods of questioning your purpose or belief system can lead to emotional stress, potentially manifesting as anxiety, insomnia, or fatigue.

Transformative Healing Through Learning

Higher education, spiritual exploration, or philosophical shifts can be healing and regenerative. Studying alternative medicine or holistic health philosophies might align with your nature.

Innovative Approaches to Wellness

Aquarius's influence suggests you may be drawn to futuristic or unconventional health practices, such as biohacking, meditation retreats, or experimental therapies.

Hidden Health Challenges

Pluto's placement can indicate hidden or slow-developing health issues. These might come to light during times of spiritual or intellectual upheaval.

Suggestions for Wellness

Expand Your Perspective

Engage in practices that align mind and body, such as mindfulness, yoga, or philosophical study. Exploring these areas can bring clarity and emotional balance, positively influencing your health.

Nervous System Support

Incorporate activities like deep breathing exercises, tai chi, or nature walks to soothe the nervous system.

Stay Grounded During Travel

When traveling, maintain routines that support physical and emotional health, such as staying hydrated, practicing regular movement, and managing stress.

Explore Holistic Healing

Embrace alternative therapies or spiritual practices that resonate with your quest for meaning, such as Reiki, acupuncture, or herbal remedies.

Challenge Limiting Beliefs

Address and transform any belief systems that restrict personal growth or contribute to stress. Journaling or speaking with a mentor or spiritual guide may help.

Physical Activity for Circulation

Regular exercise that improves circulation, such as cycling, walking, or swimming, is essential for supporting physical health, especially in the legs and ankles.

Herbs

Sage for spiritual clarity, holy basil for expansive thinking, and elderflower for resilience.

Gemstones

Lapis lazuli for wisdom, turquoise for spiritual grounding, and aventurine for exploration.

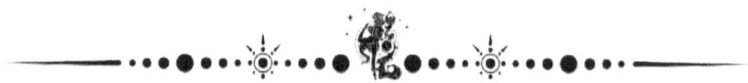

Pluto in Aquarius in the Ninth House ties your health to your beliefs, intellectual growth, and spiritual journey. Health challenges may arise during times of philosophical crisis or while navigating new experiences, but this placement offers profound regenerative potential. By expanding your mindset, embracing innovative health practices, and grounding yourself during periods of change, you can achieve a holistic sense of well-being and transformation.

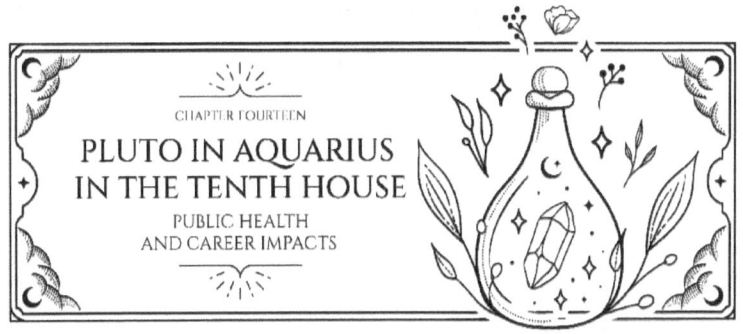

Chapter 14

Pluto in Aquarius in the Tenth House: Public Health and Career Impacts

The influence of societal roles, reputation, and career on health and well-being. Pluto in Aquarius in the Tenth House links themes of transformation, ambition, and public identity to your health and well-being. This placement suggests that career pressures, societal expectations, and personal goals significantly influence your physical and emotional health.

Pluto represents transformation, intensity, and regeneration, often demanding deep changes and fostering growth through challenges.

Aquarius, an air sign, rules the circulatory system, lower legs, ankles, and the nervous system. It is associated with innovation, detachment, and future-oriented thinking.

Tenth House (Career and Public Image)

The Tenth House governs career, public reputation, long-term goals, and authority. It also relates to how you define success and your role in the world. In terms of health, this house often reflects the impact of career stress, social status, and ambition on overall well-being.

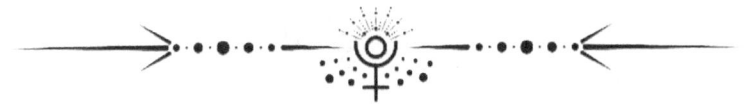

HEALTH IMPLICATIONS

Stress and Career-Driven Health Concerns

Career pressures or public responsibilities might lead to stress-related health issues, such as chronic fatigue, anxiety, or nervous system imbalances.

Circulatory and Nervous System Vulnerabilities

Aquarius's influence highlights the need for movement and relaxation to prevent poor circulation (especially in the legs and ankles) and to maintain nervous system health.

Emotional Toll of Ambition

Intense focus on achieving success or managing public image may result in emotional burnout, which can manifest physically, such as through tension headaches or sleep disturbances.

Health Issues as a Transformative Catalyst

Pluto's presence suggests that health crises tied to work or reputation may act as wake-up calls, pushing you toward healthier boundaries and habits.

Innovative Approaches to Wellness

You may be drawn to futuristic or unconventional health practices that align with your need for progress and efficiency, such as biohacking, wearable health tech, or cutting-edge treatments.

Work-Life Balance is Crucial

Pluto in the Tenth House demands a balance between ambition and self-care. Ignoring personal needs in pursuit of success could lead to health challenges.

Suggestions for Wellness

Manage Career Stress
Set boundaries around work hours and prioritize activities that relieve stress, such as meditation, exercise, or hobbies.

Physical Activity for Circulation
Regular movement, such as walking, yoga, or cycling, helps counteract the physical effects of a sedentary or overly demanding career.

Adopt Innovative Health Practices
Explore modern health solutions, such as wearable fitness trackers, advanced medical treatments, or personalized wellness programs.

Ground Yourself Emotionally
Practices like mindfulness, therapy, or journaling can help you process the emotional

toll of career pressures and maintain a balanced perspective.

Focus on Long-Term Sustainability
Cultivate habits that support your health over time, such as proper nutrition, regular exercise, and adequate rest, rather than sacrificing well-being for short-term success.

Monitor Nervous System Health
Incorporate calming practices like tai chi, breathwork, or massage therapy to maintain nervous system equilibrium, especially during high-stress periods.

Herbs
Rhodiola for stress management, peppermint for focus, and ginkgo for mental stamina.

Gemstones
Pyrite for ambition, onyx for strength, and sapphire for clarity in leadership.

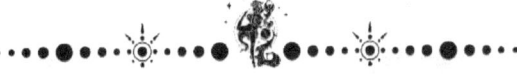

Pluto in Aquarius in the Tenth House ties your health closely to your ambitions and public life. Career pressures and the pursuit of success can affect your physical and emotional well-being, but this placement also offers the power of transformation. By maintaining work-life balance, embracing innovative health practices, and prioritizing self-care, you can achieve sustainable success and overall wellness.

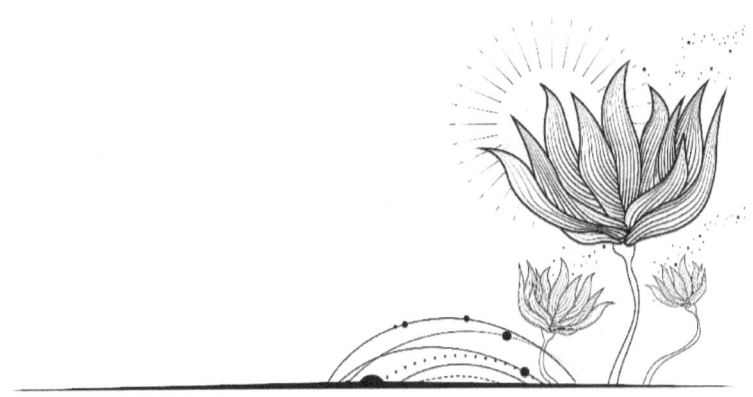

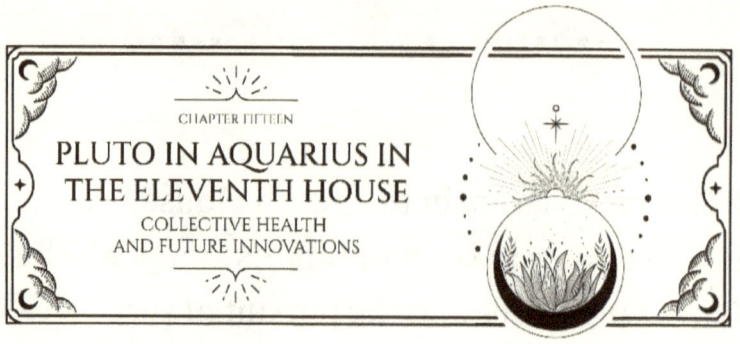

Chapter 15

Pluto in Aquarius in the Eleventh House: Collective Health and Future Innovations

Advancing group healing, technological health solutions, and community initiatives. Pluto in Aquarius in the Eleventh House, your health and well-being are deeply connected to your social networks, community involvement, and long-term aspirations. This placement emphasizes transformation through friendships, group dynamics, and your role in larger societal causes, which can influence your mental and physical health.

Pluto symbolizes transformation, intensity, and regeneration. It encourages profound changes in the areas it touches, often through deep personal challenges.

Aquarius, as an air sign, governs the circulatory system, lower legs, ankles, and the nervous system. It also represents innovative thinking, social connections, and collective progress.

Eleventh House (Community and Aspirations)

The Eleventh House governs friendships, social groups, humanitarian efforts, and long-term goals. It reflects how your relationships and ambitions in the collective sphere impact your health and well-being.

Health Implications

Impact of Social Dynamics on Health
Conflicts or challenges within friendships or social circles can create stress, which may manifest as anxiety, fatigue, or nervous system imbalances.

Circulatory and Nervous System Sensitivity
Aquarius's influence on the circulatory and nervous systems means that poor circulation or tension in the legs and ankles could be exacerbated by emotional or social stress.

Stress from Group Responsibilities
Overcommitment to social causes or group dynamics may lead to burnout, affecting your mental and physical health.

Regenerative Potential Through Community

Healing and transformation may come through positive group connections. Involvement in innovative or humanitarian projects can inspire personal growth and promote well-being.

Health Linked to Goals and Aspirations

Unrealized or overly ambitious long-term goals can cause emotional strain. Finding balance between striving for your dreams and maintaining your health is crucial.

Drawn to Futuristic Health Practices

Pluto in Aquarius suggests an affinity for unconventional or cutting-edge health approaches, such as biohacking, advanced medical technologies, or collaborative wellness programs.

Suggestions for Wellness

Manage Social Stress
Maintain boundaries within friendships and group activities to avoid emotional burnout. Learn to say no when needed.

Support the Circulatory and Nervous Systems
Engage in activities like walking, swimming, or yoga to enhance circulation and relieve tension in the nervous system.

Join Supportive Communities
Participate in positive social or wellness groups that align with your values. Community involvement can be both healing and empowering.

Pursue Balance in Goals

Break down ambitious goals into manageable steps to reduce stress and maintain motivation without overextending yourself.

Explore Innovative Health Practices

Embrace modern health technologies, alternative therapies, or collaborative wellness initiatives to enhance your overall health.

Ground Yourself Emotionally

Incorporate mindfulness practices, such as journaling or meditation, to process emotional stress tied to friendships or societal responsibilities.

Herbs

Lemon balm for social stress, astragalus for immune health, and mint for freshness in ideas.

Gemstones

Aquamarine for friendships, turquoise for community connections, and sodalite for group harmony.

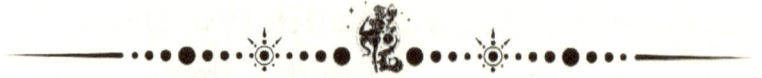

Pluto in Aquarius in the Eleventh House highlights the transformative impact of social connections and long-term aspirations on your health. While stress from group dynamics or ambitious goals can affect your well-being, this placement also provides opportunities for profound regeneration through community involvement and innovative practices. By balancing your social and personal needs, embracing modern health approaches, and fostering supportive connections, you can maintain both health and happiness.

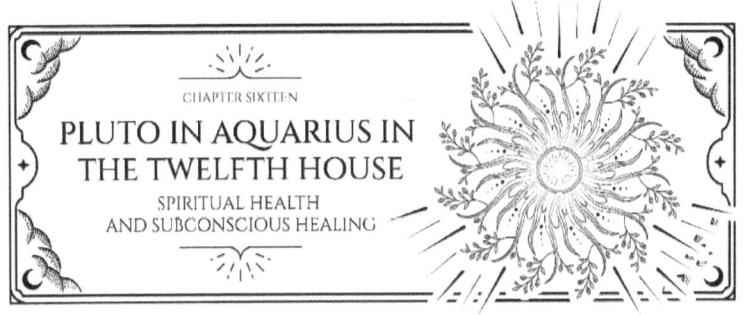

Chapter 16

Pluto in Aquarius in the Twelfth House: Spiritual Health and Subconscious Healing

Delving into the realm of solitude, mental health, and spiritual regeneration. Pluto in Aquarius in the Twelfth House, your health and well-being are deeply intertwined with your subconscious mind, spiritual growth, and hidden emotional patterns. This placement emphasizes profound transformation through introspection, healing unseen wounds, and exploring the depths of your psyche.

Pluto governs transformation, regeneration, and deep psychological processes. It often works behind the scenes, revealing hidden truths and encouraging renewal.

Aquarius, as an air sign, rules the circulatory system, lower legs, ankles, and the nervous system. It also brings a focus on innovation, detachment, and collective ideals.

Twelfth House (Subconscious and Spirituality)

The Twelfth House represents the subconscious, dreams, spiritual realms, and hidden aspects of life. It governs how unresolved emotions or karmic patterns affect your health, often pointing to psychosomatic conditions or hidden health challenges.

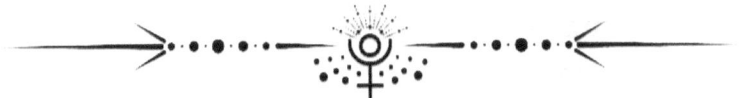

HEALTH IMPLICATIONS

Hidden or Chronic Health Issues
Pluto in the Twelfth House can indicate health issues that are difficult to diagnose or may remain hidden until triggered by emotional or spiritual crises.

Psychosomatic Symptoms
Emotional stress, unresolved traumas, or suppressed feelings may manifest physically, often affecting the nervous system or circulatory health (e.g., poor circulation, anxiety-related symptoms).

Need for Rest and Solitude
Overstimulation or lack of downtime may lead to burnout or exhaustion. Regular periods of rest and introspection are essential for maintaining health.

Transformative Healing Through Spirituality

This placement offers significant potential for healing through spiritual or introspective practices, such as meditation, dream analysis, or energy healing.

Sensitivity to Collective Energy

You may be highly sensitive to the emotions of others or the collective energy around you. This sensitivity can lead to stress or overwhelm, impacting your mental and physical health.

Drawn to Unconventional Healing Practices

Aquarius's influence suggests an attraction to innovative or unconventional health modalities, such as hypnosis, biofeedback, or holistic therapies.

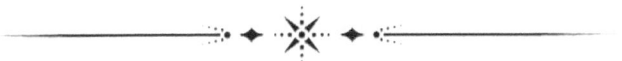

Suggestions for Wellness

Embrace Introspection and Healing
Engage in practices that allow you to explore and release subconscious blocks, such as therapy, journaling, or shadow work.

Regular Solitude and Relaxation
Schedule time for quiet reflection, meditation, or time in nature to recharge your emotional and physical energy.

Explore Dream and Subconscious Work
Pay attention to your dreams and subconscious messages. Practices like dream journaling or guided visualization can provide insights into your health.

Support the Nervous and Circulatory Systems

Incorporate calming exercises like yoga, tai chi, or deep breathing to maintain equilibrium and support circulation.

Protect Your Energy

Set boundaries to prevent absorbing negative energy from others. Practices like grounding exercises, energy clearing, or spending time alone can help.

Consider Holistic and Alternative Therapies

Explore therapies like Reiki, acupuncture, or sound healing, which resonate with the Twelfth House's connection to the unseen and spiritual realms.

Herbs

Mugwort for dream work, chamomile for spiritual rest, and ashwagandha for grounding.

Gemstones

Amethyst for spiritual insight, selenite for clearing energy, and black tourmaline for protection.

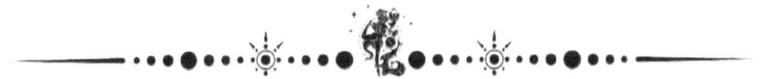

Pluto in Aquarius in the Twelfth House ties your health to the hidden and spiritual aspects of your life. Emotional and spiritual healing are key to maintaining physical well-being. While you may face hidden health challenges or psychosomatic symptoms, this placement offers profound potential for regeneration through introspection, spiritual growth, and innovative approaches to healing. By nurturing your subconscious and maintaining balance between solitude and connection, you can achieve lasting transformation and wellness.

REFERENCES

Judith Hill, *"Medical Astrology: A Guide to Planetary Pathology"* – For insights into Pluto's transformative health implications.

Richard Tarnas, *"Cosmos and Psyche: Intimations of a New World View"* – Exploring the archetypal meaning of Pluto and its societal influence.

Donna Cunningham, *"Healing Pluto Problems"* – A deep dive into the personal and collective impact of Pluto's energy.

Nick Campion, *"The Book of World Horoscopes"* – For historical context on Pluto's transit and global trends.

Barbara Hand Clow, *"Chiron: Rainbow Bridge Between the Inner and Outer Planets"* – For integrative perspectives on planetary health influences.

Urania Trust Publications – Articles and essays on astrology and health connections.

The Aquarian Age Healing Arts Directory – Contemporary holistic health practices aligned with Aquarian principles.

Astrological Journal Archives – In-depth articles on Pluto and Aquarius written by leading astrologers.

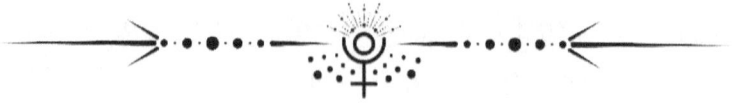

Appendix: Additional Resources and Insights

Glossary of Terms

Pluto: The planet associated with transformation, regeneration, and uncovering hidden truths.

Aquarius: A zodiac sign symbolizing innovation, community, technology, and the collective good.

Holistic Health: An approach to wellness that integrates the body, mind, and spirit.

Planetary Health: A concept emphasizing the interconnectedness of human health and the environment.

Recommended Reading

1. *"Cosmos and Psyche"* by Richard Tarnas
2. *"Healing Pluto Problems"* by Donna Cunningham
3. *"Astrology and the Rising of Kundalini"* by Barbara Hand Clow
4. *"The Only Astrology Book You'll Ever Need"* by Joanna Martine Woolfolk

Resources

Astrological Software: Tools like Solar Fire for generating detailed natal charts.

Online Courses: Astrology training programs from institutions like Kepler College and the International Academy of Astrology (IAA).

Communities: Online forums and discussion groups such as Astro.com or Astrology Weekly.

Tables and Data

Pluto's Transit Dates in Aquarius:
Initial Entry: March 23, 2023
Retrograde to Capricorn: June 11, 2023
Re-entry into Aquarius: January 20, 2024
Final Exit: January 19, 2044

Major Astrological Aspects:
Pluto square Uranus: Highlighting societal shifts and innovation.

Pluto trine Neptune: Aiding spiritual and emotional healing.

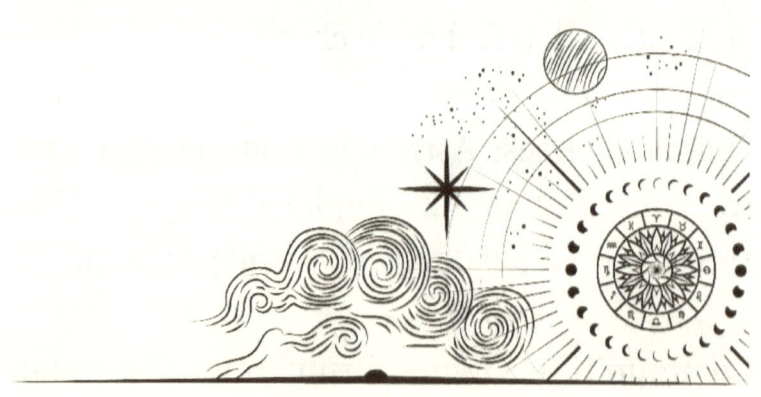

Notes for Practitioners

For medical astrologers and holistic health practitioners, understanding the interplay of Pluto and Aquarius is key to addressing issues related to stress, the nervous system, and circulatory health. Consider using techniques such as:

- Mindfulness and meditation for mental clarity.
- Herbal remedies like Ginkgo Biloba for circulation.

- Community-based health initiatives to align with Aquarian themes of collective healing.

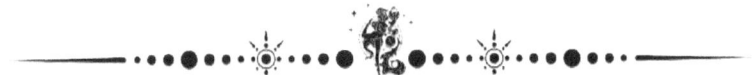

www.ingramcontent.com/pod-product-compliance
Lightning Source LLC
Chambersburg PA
CBHW031437120626
46545CB00006B/2447